SCIENCE OF HEALTHY EATING

Steven Smith

Wisdom Publishers

ISBN: 9798386691349
Imprint: Independently published

Cover design by: Art Painter
Library of Congress Control Number: 2018675309
Printed in the United States of America

To the readers who desire good health and are committed to making positive changes in their lives. This book is dedicated to you. May the Science of Healthy Eating provide you with the knowledge and tools to make informed choices and achieve your health goals. Your dedication to improving your health is an inspiration to me and many others.

Thank you for choosing to read this book and for embarking on a journey towards better health. May it be a valuable resource in your pursuit of a healthier lifestyle.

"Let food be thy medicine and medicine be thy food."

HIPPOCRATES

CONTENTS

INTRODUCTION

Welcome to the world of healthy eating! In this book, we explore the science behind eating for optimal health. With so much conflicting information about what to eat, it can be challenging to know where to start. But when we understand the science behind nutrition, we can make informed decisions about what we eat and how it affects our bodies. This book is designed to guide you through the science of healthy eating, from understanding the role of nutrients in our bodies to learning how to make healthy choices that meet your unique needs. We delve into the latest nutrition research, uncover the truth about popular diets and nutrition trends, and explore the many benefits of whole foods and natural ingredients. Whether you want to lose weight, increase your energy, or eat better, this book has something for you. We provide practical tips and recipes to help you integrate healthy eating into your everyday life. From the science of nutrition and metabolism to the benefits of superfoods, this book is your comprehensive guide to healthy eating. So let's explore the many benefits of feeding our bodies the right foods and discover how good nutrition can lead to a happier, healthier life.

For some reason, one of the hardest things for a human being is to eat right. Whether that's because we have limited access to resources or have too much access to unhealthy foods, there are many reasons why eating healthy is a challenge. Sure, we can eat almost anything, and it will nourish us. We will manage to move from one moment to the next and call ourselves healthy. But is it healthy to eat a diet of processed foods and sugary drinks? Just because we're alive doesn't mean we're healthy. And the older we get, the more our bad habits catch up. Developing healthy eating habits early in life, or at least as early as possible, is essential to prevent future problems. You don't want to wake up one day to find that you have been nutrient deficient for years, causing almost impossible complications. We all need to take more responsibility for what we put into our bodies because it can become dangerous if we don't.

When we are older and can reflect on our mistakes, hindsight is 20/20. We realize that there were things that we could have done and probably should have done that we didn't do because we were either unconscious of the ill effects or simply lazy. Just having simple knowledge does not necessarily make the need to do something health-conscious a reality. For the most part, it takes us genuinely being exposed to the suffering that can occur because of bad health choices before we are more conscious of how we treat our bodies and our health in general. When we can't see the reality of the consequences of our actions, it can make them feel very far away and difficult to relate with. We may even blow them off entirely. This can be a very debilitating place to find yourself in, especially when you are already dealing with the side effects of poor eating and a lack of a healthy diet.

Everybody deserves a chance to become the most excellent version of themselves possible. Still, we must acknowledge that unhealthy eating can take us off course, even now. In that case, we ultimately wave goodbye to the best future possible. But all of this can change. By reading this book, you will understand the importance of eating healthy and how food impacts our bodies and functions. It can sometimes be challenging to stay on track without understanding exactly why our bodies react to food the way they do. But there are many ways that you can begin to understand why eating healthy foods is so important and exactly how to begin a healthy eating journey. Let's not waste any more time. We should begin eating healthy today!

CHAPTER ONE: THE ESSENCE OF HEALTHY EATING

Healthy eating is essential for maintaining optimal health and well-being. It is about consuming a balanced diet that provides the body with the necessary nutrients and energy to function at its best. Eating healthy does not have to be complicated or restrictive; it simply means making informed food choices. The essence of healthy eating lies in consuming various nutrient-dense foods that nourish the body. This includes whole grains, fruits, vegetables, lean proteins, healthy fats, and low-fat dairy products. These foods provide a range of essential vitamins, minerals, and other nutrients that the body needs to thrive.

Most of us are already aware of the increasing obesity epidemic. This is particularly true of the United States. There is even a phrase for the way many Americans eat, and that is called the SAD diet. SAD stands for Standard American Diet, which refers to a diet low in vegetables, high in fat and sugar, and lacking in nutrition. Processed foods are a part of the SAD diet. These foods are readily available and quick to consume and prepare but have long-lasting adverse health effects. Suppose you do not want to find yourself obese. In that case, it is generally considered a good idea to avoid eating such processed foods and focus on eating whole grains, fruits and vegetables, and meat that has not been treated with hormones and other chemicals that can ultimately end up in your body and cause issues. Unfortunately, in North America, we are given a lot of options to slack off when it comes to preparing meals.

We have so many things readily available, and the money you spend to buy lousy food is far less than buying good food. It seems strange that it costs more money to buy organic than foods that will ultimately cause health problems in the long run, but that is the rule of supply and demand. Not only that, but processed foods are mass-produced and make a huge profit because of their convenience. That is why, in many ways, and obesity epidemic in North America is not particularly surprising. Nutrition is not number one on the list of companies attempting to cash in on people's laziness in the kitchen. However, in many ways eating healthy is essential and an excellent reason to avoid processed foods and the standard American diet. For example, if you do not want to be obese, you should look into the rest of this book for ways to improve your diet and begin a healthier lifestyle.

Another reason to eat healthily is that you can make yourself prone to diseases by eating unhealthy foods and staying on a standard American diet full of fat and sugar. Diabetes can be developed because of poor eating and can often be treated with healthy eating. Type II diabetes can ultimately be maintained and controlled with proper eating habits and triggered by poor eating habits. To avoid these difficulties and complications, you should do your best to be conscientious about your food choices. Other diseases can result from poor eating as well. High blood pressure is common, as well as other chronic diseases. Osteoporosis can affect many people later in life because they do not make healthy eating choices earlier. You may suffer from poor bone health, hypertension, or even heart problems. All of which can be very demanding on your body and cause significant stress that can ultimately be very dangerous.

If you want to show your family that you care about them, you should begin making choices that will help you stay in their lives for as long as possible. Poor health is not something that only affects you. It is also something that affects the people around you. If they are watching you suffer because of poor choices that you have made, in a way, that is entirely selfish. They are suffering too. Now, do your best to make the choices that will be the best not only for yourself but for your family in the long run. This book will show you how.

CHAPTER TWO: YOU AND FOOD

Over time, everybody begins to develop certain habits. We develop habits in all areas of our lives. We develop hygiene habits, food habits, work habits, and all sorts of other types of habits. However, they are oblivious to our habits until they affect us negatively. And even then, when we begin to understand that our habits poorly impact us, it can be challenging to change them. Because that is what I have, it is like. A habit is something that we do almost unconsciously. We are programmed to follow these habits; it takes tremendous willpower to break free from the cycle. Once you begin to understand that your relationship with food has everything to do with the habits that you have created and habits that you can continue to mold and cultivate, then it becomes far easier to change your mindset.

When you realize the impact and importance of your future and make positive choices about these things, it can make you more primed toward healthy eating and less inclined to make choices that negatively impact you and your future. To be truthful, many of us consider the future bleak. We need to see reasons enough to change our habits because if we believe we have something good to look forward to, it doesn't matter whether we make good choices. We do not see how we can pave our future to be in our best interests, probably because we do not have any power over our lives.

If you can relate to this feeling, don't be alarmed. It is prevalent in the human experience. We are generally discouraged from taking control and utilizing our power from an early age and sometimes stop believing we have any authority over our lives because we are usually told what to do by other people. As children, that makes sense. Children don't always know what is best for them. But it can encourage a very helpless mindset that causes us to have a hard time understanding that the consequences of our actions can truly begin to shape who we are and how we present ourselves to the world. This is why it is essential to truly take steps to help you understand yourself and your dietary habits. When did your habit begin? How did you form that habit? Why? What benefits do you have from this habit? What adverse effects do you have from this habit?

Ask yourself as many of these questions as you can so that you begin to have indeed an understanding of how it is that you are shaping your future with the food that you are eating. Are you creating a healthy and energized future, or are you creating a bleak one that is potentially full of adverse health consequences? Next, evaluate your sense of self-discipline. Are you capable of maintaining discipline over your choices? Or is this an area where you struggle? Discipline can be difficult for everybody, and if you find yourself having difficulty staying disciplined, it will do you well to look into different ways to encourage yourself to be a more disciplined person both in practice and mentally.

Only then will you have what it takes to begin a healthy eating journey. Because whether we like it or not, bad health choices are everywhere. They are easy, and they are addicting. If we allow ourselves to be swayed by these poor choices and do nothing to change our habits, then it doesn't matter whether you eat healthy sometimes or not. The adverse effects will still be gripping your body and waiting to spring up on you when you least expect them. In a way, unhealthy eating is a self-destructive pattern unknowingly to many. Whether this is because of poor self-esteem or simply because we are unhappy with our situations and have no faith in the future, self-destructive eating patterns are dangerous. You must look to yourself and truly value your life and future before eating healthy will stick. You can do this in many ways and may even want to consult a mental health professional for support. Sometimes, they help us to see biases and negative patterns in our lives that we remain oblivious to. Once those are understood and accepted, it can be much easier to overcome them and take the steps you need to take to make positive choices.

Whether you seek out the help of a qualified professional or not, there are many things that you can do to change your mindset. If you understand that you are worthy of a healthy body and a positive future, you will allow yourself to take the steps necessary to get there. But it will be a lot harder if you do not feel good about yourself. Understanding yourself, habits, mental roadblocks, and discipline will help you. We can take steps every day toward becoming our best possible selves, and healthy eating is one significant step in that direction. And it is a step we can take today!

CHAPTER THREE: DIETING MENACE

Dieting restricts food intake to achieve a desired body weight and shape. While dieting can lead to short-term weight loss, it can also negatively affect an individual's physical and mental health. Nutritional deficiencies, slower metabolism, eating disorders, increased risk of chronic diseases, and psychological consequences are just a few ways dieting can become a menace. Instead of resorting to restrictive or fad diets, focusing on developing a healthy diet and lifestyle, incorporating balance and moderation, and incorporating physical activity is crucial. Diet trends are rampant today, and almost all come with dangers. Unfortunately, most people desperate to make money often don't look at the long-term health consequences of their products. They are genuinely concerned about making money and doing something that will help them capitalize off of a desperate desire that many people have to lose weight quickly and easily. There is something that you are going to have to accept if diet trends are something that captivates your interest. Unfortunately, there is no healthy way to lose weight fast and quickly with no work, healthy eating, or exercise. Losing weight is a good goal if you are obese or lacking in fitness and need extra mobility.

All of us have, at times, needed to start making better lifestyle choices, and that is something that we can do with food and healthy body movement instead of trusting companies that want to exploit us to make money. Some diet trends are dangerous and have dire health consequences, both long-term and short-term. Many rely on methods that cause us to starve our bodies of essential nutrients. Sometimes even dehydrating us. These types of diet trends are highly disgusting. They are taking advantage of people who want to be healthy but don't know how to do it. They are taking advantage of people, often women in particular, who are crumbling under the pressures of unrealistic beauty standards and women who are told that to have any value, they must look a certain way. That is untrue. Whether you weigh 100 pounds or 700 pounds, you have value. However, healthy eating is one of the only natural ways that you are going to be able to kickstart your metabolism and provide your body with the nutrients that it needs to function at its highest possible capacity.

If you are robbing your body of the vitamins and minerals it needs to thrive and trusting a diet trend to teach you how to lose weight and have value when all they want is your money, you will end up further behind the line. The unfortunate truth about many diet trends is that they cause the body to go into starvation mode. This can wreck your metabolism and cause you to gain weight even faster in the future. Don't let yourself be exploited by advertisements promising that you will lose weight quickly and easily. All of that will come with a price. Also, there are health trends, such as the hCG diet, that can screw up your body and hormones. The ironic thing about diet trends is that they often will make it harder for you to lose weight in the future because you are implementing unhealthy and challenging ways of maintaining your weight. If you want to be skinny, don't trust a pill on TV to make you skinny. Start cutting out unhealthy sugary, and processed foods and replace them with healthy whole-grain wheat and organic fruits and vegetables that will not introduce chemicals into your body that will make it even harder for you to lose weight and that will ultimately mess up your body chemistry.

It may seem tempting to be able to lose weight quickly and not have to sacrifice the negative eating habits that you have developed over your lifetime, but it is not healthy. You are hurting yourself and priming your body for further health complications if you are not careful about how you attempt to lose weight. Make sure you are doing everything in your power to make choices that you want others to make for themselves. Research before you let yourself be swayed by the snake oil salesman on TV. Look into these things because you are worth doing things the right way, and you deserve a positive future, not one complicated by the side effects of a sales pitch that only wants your money and not your health.

CHAPTER FOUR: ORDER OF FOOD

Most of us have seen the food pyramid. Growing up, the food pyramid was often used as a guideline to provide us with an idea of how much food and what kind of food we should eat every day to maintain a healthy lifestyle. Of course, there is always evidence that the food pyramid is flexible. Still, if you can observe the food pyramid, you will have a general idea of what is acceptable in a healthy and nutritious diet. While this may sometimes be controversial, it is still good to have basic food. Possibly one that you create yourself. A lot of people will say that it is no longer considered the most healthy thing to do to eat as many grains as the food pyramid may have suggested.

Many people now rely on the food pyramid for their basic guidelines of what is healthy to eat. Try to consider your personal experiences with food and go from there. Some people are healthier with many grains, and some are not. Use your judgment here to the best of your ability so that you can take steps in the right direction for your health. The standard food pyramid recommends as follows:

- Rice, cereal, pasta, and bread can be as many as 11 servings daily.
- For vegetables and fruits, you should have between three

and five servings.

- As far as their eggs, you can have two or three servings daily, provided you are not allergic or lactose intolerant.
- When it comes to meat and beans, and other things like nuts and fish or poultry, it is recommended that you have two or three servings every day.
- Unsurprisingly, sugar, fat, and oil are the very tip of the. Because you should not have any of these things in excess. Instead, use them only as necessary to guarantee your healthiest possible lifestyle.

Again, this is only referencing the standard food pyramid. Depending on your particular needs and dietary functions, you may need to modify this order yourself. But if you do not have any specific requirements, this is the standard food order that can be utilized to your most significant possible advantage in creating a healthier lifestyle.

The food pyramid above is a visual tool that helps to guide individuals toward a healthy and balanced diet. The pyramid is divided into different food groups, each with its recommended serving sizes and types of foods. By following the recommendations on the food pyramid, individuals can reap numerous benefits for their health and well-being. One of the key benefits of following the food pyramid is that it promotes a balanced diet. The pyramid recommends consuming various foods from all food groups, including fruits, vegetables, grains, protein sources, and dairy. By including various foods in one's diet, individuals can ensure they get all the necessary nutrients for optimal health. Eating a balanced diet can also help prevent nutrient deficiencies, which can lead to various health problems.

Another benefit of the food pyramid is that it can help individuals manage their weight. The pyramid emphasizes the importance of portion control and moderation, which can help individuals maintain a healthy weight or achieve weight loss goals. By following the recommended serving sizes, individuals can prevent overeating and consume the appropriate calories for their age, gender, and activity level. Following the food pyramid can also reduce the risk of chronic diseases such as heart disease, diabetes, and cancer. This is because the recommended foods can help maintain healthy cholesterol levels, blood sugar levels, and overall health. For example, consuming a diet high in fruits and vegetables has been linked to a reduced risk of chronic diseases.

The food pyramid can also guide individuals with special dietary requirements, such as lactose intolerance or gluten sensitivities. By following the recommendations on the pyramid, individuals can ensure that they are consuming all the necessary nutrients, even if they have to modify their diet. It also serves as an educational tool for individuals of all ages. By teaching individuals about the different food groups and the importance of a balanced diet, the pyramid can help to promote healthy eating habits that can last a lifetime.

CHAPTER FIVE: MAKE FOOD YOUR MEDICINE

Make food your medicine is a well-known adage emphasizing the importance of consuming nutrient-dense foods to promote health and prevent disease. The idea that food can have a powerful impact on health has been around for centuries. Still, it has only recently gained significant attention in the medical community. The concept of food as medicine is based on the idea that the nutrients and bioactive compounds found in whole foods can have powerful health-promoting effects. By consuming a diet rich in fruits, vegetables, whole grains, lean proteins, and healthy fats, individuals can provide their bodies with the nutrients and compounds needed for optimal health.

One of the critical ways food can be used as medicine is by preventing chronic diseases. Chronic diseases, such as heart disease, diabetes, and cancer, are responsible for most deaths worldwide. However, research has shown that dietary interventions can prevent or manage many of these diseases. For example, consuming a diet high in fruits and vegetables has reduced the risk of heart disease and cancer. Food can also be used to manage existing health conditions. For example, individuals with diabetes can benefit from consuming a diet rich in complex carbohydrates, fiber, and lean proteins, as these nutrients can help to stabilize blood sugar levels. Similarly, individuals with high blood pressure may benefit from consuming a diet low in sodium and high in potassium, as this can help to regulate blood pressure levels.

The benefits of using food as medicine are not limited to physical health. Diet can also influence mental health, as certain nutrients and compounds have been shown to impact mood and cognition positively. For example, consuming omega-3 fatty acids found in fatty fish, nuts, and seeds has been linked to improved mental health outcomes, including a reduced risk of depression. It is important to note that not all foods are created equal regarding their health-promoting effects. Processed foods, high in added sugars and unhealthy fats, can negatively impact health and should be limited or avoided. Instead, individuals should focus on consuming whole, nutrient-dense foods that provide the body with the necessary nutrients for optimal health. Another critical aspect of using food as medicine is that it can be a cost-effective and accessible way to promote health. Unlike medications, which can be expensive and have potential side effects, food is widely available and affordable when chosen wisely. Additionally, incorporating healthy foods into one's diet can positively impact overall health, reducing the need for costly medical interventions in the future.

In the same way that not eating healthy can make you sick, eating healthy foods can frequently cure you of illness and relieve you when you are suffering. It can also act as a preventative measure to take against illness. There has been an entire healing method around India for thousands of years called Aryuveda. This ancient healing style treats any illness simply by changing your diet. Food is the medicine that has helped to keep the people of India alive for centuries. And it can still be applicable today. Many remedies are healthy foods with anti-inflammatory properties and can nourish your body from the inside out. Healthy eating choices have impacted everything from infection to cancer. And with this ancient healing art, that has never been more apparent.

Of course, much modern technology will frown upon these methods because they have yet to be scientifically investigated. Still, it has been tried and true for thousands of years and will continue to impact the body. Whether you believe in the ancient healing art or not, the fact remains that food can ultimately determine whether or not you are susceptible to illness. If you eat well, your body will be stronger, and it will be able to fight off illness and infection far easier than it would if you find yourself malnourished on the standard American diet. Without the proper vitamins and minerals in your body, fighting off the adverse effects of illness can be almost impossible. Sometimes, it can even cause illness. If you are eating unhealthy unprocessed foods, certain foods can lead to illnesses and make you more susceptible to certain types of cancer.

Although cancer is still being researched and has not been fully understood by the scientific community well enough to cure it, many people could live long and healthy lives simply by changing the way they need it. Healthy eating can help decrease the symptoms of many complex and impossible-to-cure diseases, such as multiple sclerosis. As long as you ensure that everything you put into your body is nourishing and provides your organs and cells with all of the fuel and resources they need to keep your body strong, they will continue to do that. And they will do it to the best of their ability. However, if you are actively sabotaging your body, they will not be able to put up the same fight as they would if they were receiving adequate nutrition. That is why it is so vital for you to take heed of the way you are nourishing your body. If you are not making active and conscientious choices about your food, you could be setting yourself up for failure in ways that you may live to regret.

CHAPTER SIX: VEGETABLE HEALTH BENEFITS

Vegetables are one of the most under-sung foods in existence, especially when it comes to the standard American diet. Most people need to realize just how important it is to provide the body with the vitamins and minerals that vegetables and vegetables alone can provide. Sometimes, people will look into vegetables to improve their beauty, but when it comes to improving their health, they become somewhat disinterested. However, now that you are here and reading this book, it is safe to assume that you are willing and able to consider why it is important to eat vegetables. Here are some of the best reasons to provide yourself with vegetables daily.

First of all, the body needs fiber to get rid of excess waste. Without a way to find the waste together and eliminate it, it stays stuck in the body and can contribute to weight gain and other potential complications. Fiber is essential for other reasons as well. It can help you prevent your blood cholesterol from rising and even prevent heart disease, or at least lower the chances of suffering from it. Folic acid is also present in vegetables; when you provide your body with this substance, it can produce red blood cells. This can be very important in helping you prevent anemia and can be very beneficial to women, in particular, who tend to need this substance during pregnancy and menstruation.

Vegetables are also naturally high in many vitamins, such as a and C, which help fight infection and keep the body healthy. It can help you speed up the healing process and absorb iron, which is another way of helping combat and prevents anemia. Vitamins are high in potassium, which is helpful because it prevents the body from succumbing to high blood pressure. Vegetables have been proven to reduce the risk of strokes and other heart-related complications. They can prevent kidney stones from developing and disintegrating bone matter. Filling yourself with vegetables is an excellent way to help you manage type II diabetes and obesity.

Not only that, but it can help you stay strong in the fight against cancer and cancer prevention. One of the most redeeming qualities of eating vegetables is that they are deficient in fat and are not calorie-dense. This means you can eat as many vegetables as you want without worrying too much about gaining weight. Snacking on vegetables is a great way to help you to reduce hunger cravings and to stay focused on a healthy lifestyle. There are so many great things about vegetables. Surprisingly, they are so rare in the standard American diet. One of the best ways to help yourself avoid high-fat, high-sugar, and high-salt processed foods is by first walking around the outside of your grocery store.

Go along the fresh produce section to make conscious choices in providing your body with healthy fresh vegetable options rather than skipping to the end and cheating by buying pasta and other processed foods that are low in nutritional vegetable content. Healthy eating starts with choosing to nourish your body, and there are few things more nourishing than vegetables. We can often lose our taste for healthy foods because of unhealthy and poor eating habits early in life or even self-imposed later in life, but it is easy to get back on track. Make time in your life for vegetables. They may take longer to prepare, but the benefits are worth it.

CHAPTER SEVEN: FRUITS' HEALTH BENEFITS

It is unfortunate but common knowledge that people who follow the standard American diet do not eat enough fruit. What fruit they eat is usually found in cans or saturated with sugar. The added sugar and fruit are something that takes away any health benefits that eating fruit in its natural state can provide the body. Overeating fruit can have some complications, especially if you have diabetes. Fruit is high in natural sugars, and when it is juiced, you get a lot of sugar without a lot of fiber, which can give the body an excess. The fiber present in fruits is one of the things that makes them the healthiest and helps the body lower heart disease and avoid constipation. Not only that, but fiber-rich foods like fruit and vegetables are very beneficial for weight management because it helps you to feel full with fewer calories. Not only that, but fruits are high in many vitamins and minerals, especially citrus fruits when it comes to vitamin C. Vitamin C is a powerhouse for helping the body heal. Vitamin C-rich fruits will do the trick if you need something that will help keep your teeth and gums healthy.

Another thing fruit can help the body achieve stroke and kidney stone prevention. Fruits are very helpful in supporting the body and preventing and fighting disorders such as skin conditions and heart problems. Fruit can be one of the most healthy ways to help you boost energy and get rid of sugar cravings that you may have when attempting to cut unhealthy foods out of your diet. As long as you aren't overdoing it with your fruits, such as throwing a bunch of them in the blender and ultimately consuming a ridiculous amount of sugar, then you can have a healthy snack that satisfies your sweet tooth if you are willing to utilize the tremendous power of fruit.

If you are interested in the benefits of food to your health, both fruits and vegetables naturally tend to help your skin glow and appear far more hydrated and nourished. Fruits and vegetables are high in antioxidants, vitamins, and minerals that provide your body with the hydration necessary to keep your skin and appearance healthy. It can help your hair grow softer and healthier, as well as retain the youthful look of your skin. Fruit can even help you stop acne by keeping your body free of waste products that come out through your pores and hydrating your skin. Fruit is excellent for helping the body stay hydrated because of its high water content, and you will quickly begin to see the benefits.

Not only that, but the fruit is beneficial for digestion. Because of the high fiber content, it helps to bind waste and helps the body eliminate things that might otherwise cause issues. Because of this, fruit and vegetables can also aid in weight loss. Rather than allowing waste to be broken down and stored as fat, the body eliminates it before it has the chance. Fruit is another great way to help you to fight and prevent disease, even cancer. Some fruits, such as apples, help to keep asthma at bay. Others can significantly lower cholesterol levels.

Grapes have been known to be used in the combat of cancer, particularly red-skinned grapes. They are also helpful in fighting eye issues and kidney problems. If you suffer from infection, berries are beneficial. They are high in antioxidants. Just make sure you are eating fruits and vegetables that are not treated with commercial pesticides, as they can absorb these chemicals and complicate weight loss and cause issues in the body. You can even eat dry fruits to substitute unhealthy and sugary snacks and provide your body with a sweet snack that will pack quite a nutritional punch. Just be conscientious of the sugar levels in dried fruits because sometimes, when they are commercially sold, added sugars make a healthy treat into something that may ultimately help you pack on the pounds. However, when you are eating fruit in a healthy way, and regularly, fruit can help you lose weight. As long as you are not overeating things high in sugar, the fibers and water content of fruit will help your body feel full and nourish your cells and organs. The fibers and water content will help you eliminate issues contributing to obesity, and overall you will feel an immense shift in your energy levels. You can utilize this energy to exercise and work harder toward a healthy lifestyle. This can be especially effective if you replace sugary junk foods with healthier fruit alternatives as you continue to transition toward better health and well-being.

CHAPTER EIGHT: GRAINS HEALTH BENEFITS

Grains are an essential food group that is commonly consumed worldwide. They include wheat, barley, rice, corn, oats, millet, and others. Grains are an excellent source of carbohydrates, fiber, vitamins, and minerals. They are a crucial component of a healthy diet and offer numerous health benefits when consumed in the right quantities. This chapter will discuss the benefits of eating grains, the different types available, and how to incorporate them into your diet for optimal health.

Good for Digestion

Grains are a rich source of dietary fiber, which plays a vital role in maintaining digestive health. Fiber helps to prevent constipation, reduce the risk of diverticulitis, and promote the growth of healthy gut bacteria. Whole grains, in particular, contain insoluble fiber, which adds bulk to the stool and promotes regular bowel movements.

Promotes Heart Health

Grains are also beneficial for heart health. Studies have shown that consuming whole grains can help lower the risk of heart disease, stroke, and high blood pressure. This is because whole grains contain antioxidants, fiber, and other nutrients that help to reduce inflammation and improve blood flow. The fiber in whole grains also helps lower cholesterol levels, a significant risk factor for heart disease.

Helps with Weight Management

Grains are an excellent food choice for weight management. They are low in fat and calories and high in fiber, which helps to keep you feeling full for longer. This means that you are less likely to overeat or snack between meals, which can lead to weight gain. Whole grains are also a low glycemic index food, meaning they do not cause spikes in blood sugar levels, making them a good option for people with diabetes or those at risk of developing diabetes.

Provides Energy

Grains are an excellent source of carbohydrates, the body's primary energy source. Carbohydrates are broken down into glucose, which is used to fuel the body's cells. Consuming grains can help to boost energy levels and improve physical performance. Whole grains are an excellent option as they are a slow-release carbohydrate, providing sustained energy over an extended period.

Good for Brain Health

Grains are also beneficial for brain health. They contain vitamins and minerals such as B vitamins, iron, and zinc, essential for brain function. B vitamins, in particular, play a vital role in producing neurotransmitters, chemicals that transmit signals between nerve cells in the brain. Iron is also essential for brain function as it helps to carry oxygen to the brain.

May Help Prevent Cancer

Grains may also have cancer-fighting properties. Whole grains contain phytochemicals, compounds found in plant-based foods that have been shown to have anticancer properties. Phytochemicals have been shown to inhibit the growth of cancer cells and reduce the risk of certain types of cancer, including colon and breast cancer.

Types of Grains

There are two main types of grains: whole grains and refined grains. Whole grains contain the entire grain kernel, including the bran, germ, and endosperm. Examples of whole grains include brown rice, quinoa, whole wheat, and oats. Refined grains, on the other hand, have had the bran and germ removed during processing, leaving only the endosperm. Examples of refined grains include white rice, white bread, and pasta.

While both types of grains offer health benefits, whole grains are generally considered healthier. They contain more fiber, vitamins, and minerals than refined grains. Whole grains also have a lower glycemic index, meaning they do not cause blood sugar spikes like refined grains. When choosing grains, opting for whole-grain products whenever possible is essential.

How to Incorporate Grains into Your Diet

Incorporating grains into your diet is easy and can be done in various ways. Here are a few tips on how to do so:

- Swap white bread and pasta for whole-grain varieties.
- Choose brown rice instead of white rice.
- Snack on whole grain crackers or popcorn instead of chips.
- Add quinoa or brown rice to salads.
- Use whole-grain flour instead of white flour when baking.
- Try new grains like bulgur, barley, or farro.

- Make your granola or muesli using whole-grain oats.

Grains are an essential food group that offers numerous health benefits when consumed as part of a healthy diet. They are a rich source of carbohydrates, fiber, vitamins, and minerals for good health. Consuming whole grains, in particular, can help to improve digestive health, promote heart health, aid in weight management, provide energy, boost brain function, and may even help to prevent certain types of cancer. By incorporating more whole grains into your diet, you can reap the many health benefits they offer while enjoying delicious and nutritious meals.

CHAPTER NINE:
LEAN PROTEINS

Lean proteins are a protein that is low in fat and calories. They are typically found in animal sources such as poultry, fish, lean cuts of beef or pork, and plant-based sources such as beans, lentils, and tofu. Lean proteins contain all of the essential amino acids that the body needs for the growth, repair, and maintenance of tissues without the added fat and calories that can come from consuming high-fat animal proteins like bacon, sausage, or fatty cuts of meat. Some examples of lean proteins include skinless chicken breast, turkey breast, fish like salmon or tuna, and plant-based sources like soybeans, lentils, or quinoa. Incorporating lean proteins into a healthy diet can help to promote overall health and well-being. Proteins are essential macronutrients the body requires for tissue growth, repair, and maintenance. They comprise building blocks called amino acids, crucial for the body's metabolic functions. Lean proteins, in particular, are an excellent source of high-quality protein that provides various health benefits. In this chapter, we will consider the health benefits of lean proteins and some potential dangers associated with their consumption.

Health Benefits of Lean Proteins

Muscle Building and Repair

Learn proteins are an excellent source of high-quality protein essential for muscle building and repair. They contain all the necessary amino acids that the body needs to build and maintain muscle tissue. Consuming lean proteins can help increase muscle mass and improve muscle function, leading to better overall health and physical performance.

Weight Management

Consuming lean proteins can help to manage weight by increasing satiety and reducing hunger. Protein takes longer to digest than carbohydrates or fats, keeping you full longer. This can help to prevent overeating and snacking between meals, leading to a reduction in overall calorie intake and weight loss.

Improved Heart Health

Learn proteins, such as fish, chicken, and turkey, are low in saturated fats and cholesterol, which makes them an excellent choice for heart health. Research has shown that consuming lean proteins can help to lower blood pressure, reduce the risk of heart disease, and improve overall cardiovascular health.

Better Bone Health

Learn proteins are rich in calcium and other essential minerals for healthy bones. Consuming lean proteins, significantly low in fat, can help improve bone density and reduce the risk of osteoporosis.

Improved Brain Function

Proteins are essential for producing neurotransmitters, which are critical for brain function. Consuming lean proteins can help to improve cognitive function, memory, and mood. They can also help to reduce the risk of age-related cognitive decline and dementia.

Dangers of Lean Proteins

While lean proteins offer numerous health benefits, there are also potential dangers associated with their consumption. Here are some of the most significant dangers to be aware of:

Increased Risk of Kidney Disease

Consuming too much protein can increase the kidney workload and lead to kidney disease. People with pre-existing kidney disease or those at risk of developing it should be particularly cautious about their protein intake.

High-Calorie Intake

Learn proteins are often served with high-fat accompaniments such as cheese or cream sauces, which can lead to a high-calorie intake. Consuming excessive calories can lead to weight gain and other associated health problems.

Risk of Foodborne Illness

Consuming undercooked or raw lean proteins can increase the risk of foodborne illness. Proper cooking and storing of lean proteins are essential to prevent the growth of harmful bacteria that can cause illness.

Allergies

Some people may have allergies or intolerances to certain types of lean proteins, such as shellfish, fish, or poultry. It is essential to be aware of any food allergies or intolerances and avoid consuming foods that may cause an allergic reaction.

Learn proteins are an excellent source of high-quality protein with numerous health benefits. They are essential for muscle building and repair, weight management, improved heart health, better bone health, and improved brain function. However, it is essential to be aware of the potential dangers associated with their consumption, such as an increased risk of kidney disease, high-calorie intake, foodborne illness, and allergies. By consuming lean proteins in moderation and taking appropriate precautions, you can enjoy their many health benefits while minimizing associated risks.

CHAPTER TEN: HEALTHY FAT

There are two main types of healthy fats: monounsaturated and polyunsaturated fats. Monounsaturated fats are found in foods such as olive oil, avocado, nuts, and seeds, while polyunsaturated fats are found in fatty fish such as salmon, nuts, and seeds. Other sources of healthy fats include nuts and seeds such as almonds, walnuts, and chia seeds. These foods contain a range of healthy fats and other nutrients such as fiber and protein, making them a nutritious addition to a healthy diet.

Healthy fats play a role in promoting heart health. While saturated and trans fats have been linked to an increased risk of heart disease, consuming healthy fats can have the opposite effect. For example, consuming monounsaturated fats in foods such as olive oil, avocado, and nuts has improved cholesterol levels and reduced the risk of heart disease. In addition to promoting heart health, healthy fats can also have a positive impact on brain function. Omega-3 fatty acids, in particular, have been linked to improved cognitive function and a reduced risk of cognitive decline. This is because omega-3s play a crucial role in the structure and function of the brain. Healthy fats can also play a role in weight management. While fats are often associated with weight gain, eating healthy fats in moderation can promote weight loss. This is because healthy fats can increase feelings of fullness and reduce cravings for unhealthy foods. Additionally, consuming healthy fats can help to regulate blood sugar levels, reducing the risk of insulin resistance and diabetes.

However, consuming healthy fats in moderation is essential, as excessive consumption can have adverse health outcomes. Consuming too many calories from any source can lead to weight gain and an increased risk of chronic diseases. Additionally, while healthy fats have been shown to have anti-inflammatory effects, excessive consumption can lead to inflammation in the body. This is because all fats, including healthy fats, contain many calories, and consuming too many calories can lead to excess inflammation in the body. Another potential danger of consuming healthy fats is the potential for exposure to environmental toxins. Some types of fish, such as tuna and swordfish, contain high levels of mercury, which can harm health. It is important to choose fish low in mercury, such as salmon, and to consume fish in moderation to reduce the risk of exposure to environmental toxins. Consuming healthy fats in moderation is crucial to avoid adverse health outcomes such as excessive calorie consumption and inflammation. Additionally, choosing sources of healthy fats that are low in environmental toxins is essential to promote overall health and well-being.

CHAPTER ELEVEN: LOW-FAT DAIRY PRODUCTS

Low-fat dairy products are dairy products that have had some or all of the fat content removed. This can include skim, low-fat, and reduced-fat cheese, among others. Skim milk, also known as fat-free milk, has removed all creams, leaving it with less than 0.5% fat. On the other hand, low-fat milk contains slightly more fat than skim milk, typically around 1-2% fat. Reduced-fat cheese is another example of a low-fat dairy product. It contains less fat than regular cheese, typically around 25-30% less. Other low-fat dairy products include low-fat yogurt, which typically contains 2% or less fat, and low-fat cottage cheese, which typically contains around 1% fat. It is important to note that while low-fat dairy products may contain less fat than full-fat dairy products, they still contain essential nutrients such as calcium, protein, and vitamin D. These nutrients are essential for overall health and should not be overlooked when choosing low-fat dairy products.

Low-fat dairy products have become increasingly popular due to their potential health benefits. Dairy products are an important source of calcium, vitamin D, and other essential nutrients. Still, they can also be high in saturated fat, which is linked to an increased risk of heart disease and other chronic diseases. Low-fat dairy products are a way to enjoy the nutritional benefits of dairy while reducing saturated fat intake. One of the main benefits of low-fat dairy products is their potential to improve heart health. High levels of saturated fat in the diet have been linked to an increased risk of heart disease, and reducing saturated fat intake can help lower cholesterol levels and decrease the risk of heart disease. Low-fat dairy products are a good source of calcium and other essential nutrients without the excess saturated fat found in full-fat dairy products. Studies have shown that low-fat dairy products may help reduce blood pressure and improve overall heart health.

In addition to their potential heart health benefits, low-fat dairy products may also positively impact weight management. Dairy products have been shown to help with weight loss and weight management, and low-fat dairy products may be particularly effective. One study found that individuals who consumed low-fat dairy products as part of a calorie-restricted diet lost more weight and body fat than those who consumed full-fat dairy products. Another potential benefit of low-fat dairy products is their impact on bone health. Dairy products are a vital calcium source for strong bones and teeth. Low-fat dairy products can provide significant calcium without the excess calories and saturated fat found in full-fat dairy products. Additionally, low-fat dairy products are often fortified with vitamin D, essential for calcium absorption and bone health.

Despite their potential benefits, it is crucial to be mindful of the potential dangers of low-fat dairy products. Some low-fat dairy products may contain added sugars to improve taste and texture, which can contribute to excess calorie intake and adverse health outcomes. It is important to choose low-fat dairy products that are minimally processed and do not contain added sugars. Additionally, some individuals may have difficulty tolerating dairy products due to lactose intolerance or other digestive issues. In these cases, choosing alternative sources of calcium and other essential nutrients may be necessary.

CHAPTER TWELVE:
THE BEST MEAT FOR HEALTHY LIVING

Meat is generally considered one of the primary staple foods in an email, but it may be surprising that some meats are healthier than others. Of course, we know the difference between red meats and white meats. Red meats are often linked to health problems and coronary issues, while white meats are leaner and healthier overall. What some people may be surprised to find is that other issues make meats unhealthy. Issues include what they are fed while the animals are still alive and antibiotics and hormones that may be injected into them to make them grow faster or produce more milk, at least in the case of cows. These hormones ultimately enter the meat we consume and can cause problems in our bodies. Suppose we need to be more conscientious of our choices when choosing our foods. In that case, they can ultimately contribute to poor health in the future, including but not limited to cancers and hormone changes that can be pretty debilitating.

However, if you are confident that you are receiving your meat from healthy sources and do not feed animals in excess of steroids and antibiotics, then you are already ahead of the game. If not, try to research local places where you can receive meat untainted by some dangerous industry standards.

That said, even considering the healthy meat options, certain meats are healthier than others. One of the healthiest meats you can eat, especially if you hope to lose weight, is fish. Fish is lean and packed with nutrients. However, you have to be careful about the source of your fish. Some fish is raised in unhealthy conditions, while others may come from areas contaminated with mercury. This is why it is frowned upon for pregnant women to eat fish or shellfish. But if you find a healthy source of fish, this can be very beneficial for your body. Fish is high in omega-3 fatty acids, which help brain function and memory. Overall, Omega threes are highly coveted, and the body needs them to function at their highest possible potential, especially regarding intellectual matters.

Chicken that has been raised in a suitable environment is another great option. Chicken is high in protein. It is the highest in the protein of any other meat. They are usually raised in good conditions or at least fed foods that will not cause the human body issues the same way a lot of beef can. However, if you are eating grass that beef from a trustworthy supplier, that can also be a great option. If you eat organic chicken, these animals are generally less likely to be raised with dangerous carcinogens. Chickens that have been conventionally grown are usually fed foods that increase the rate at which they grow, which can lead to serious health problems for the chickens and the humans that consume them. They are also given great antidepressants, painkillers, and sometimes arsenic and caffeine. Consuming a lot of conventionally grown meat is dangerous, but if you can find a good supplier, you definitely should do so.

Turkey is another excellent meat because it is high in selenium. This is great for the body because it can help eliminate free radicals and other toxic substances. Again, you want to try to ensure that you are receiving your meat from trustworthy sources because it is standard for conventionally grown chicken and turkey to be treated similarly and fed dangerous chemicals that unnaturally increase their growth rate and contaminate human bodies with those chemicals. Eating meat can benefit the body if you are not eating meat from dangerous and conventionally grown methods. The chemicals that these animals are often subject to are exceptionally dangerous, both to the animals themselves and the humans who consume them. If you want to eat healthily and lose weight, it is better to avoid any chemicals that may end up staying stuck in your body and preventing weight loss from occurring.

Even if you are not hoping to lose weight, eating healthy includes avoiding anything that could be dangerous to the body, such as the hormones and chemicals that are disruptive to our sensitive systems. Fortunately, there are many sources for healthy meats, whether you want to indulge in chicken, beef, or even lamb. There are ways that you can get healthy, ethically raised me to satisfy any cravings you may have.

CHAPTER THIRTEEN: THE RISKS OF PROCESSED FOODS

It does not come as a surprise to anybody that processed foods are dangerous. However, it does come as a surprise that they are still allowed out on the shelves, despite the havoc they wreak on our bodies and minds. Eating unhealthy food isn't just a personal choice for some people. Sometimes, because of how the economy works, people in poverty are forced to turn to processed foods because they are a cheap and easy way to feed large families on a low budget. The tricky thing about that is that these foods ultimately cause medical problems down the line that cost even more money than it would take to feed a large family healthy, sustainable options. Ultimately, people with little money are suffering either way.

Even if you don't have to feed a family on a budget, processed foods are unhealthy. Part of what makes them so addicting is their high fat and sugar content. They often have boxed meals that include pasta and an exceptional amount of sugar. Excessive sugar is generally dangerous, but especially to people prone to developing type II diabetes. If you consume sugar and high amounts, you will ultimately overload your body, and not only will you become obese, more than likely, but you will also develop health issues. Sugar can help speed along the process of diabetes because it causes insulin resistance, which ultimately makes it difficult, if not impossible, to control your blood sugar levels. If you eat foods like this excessively, such as for every meal or at least every day, there is bound to be a negative consequence. Consuming that high amount of fat and sugar consistently can lead to not only diabetes and obesity, which are commonly known, but also heart disease and even cancer. This is exceptionally dangerous, and if possible, processed foods should be avoided at all costs.

Another danger of eating processed foods is that not only are they addicting, but they are highly artificial. Most of the ingredients in those foods are not nourishing the body. Instead, they lead us to feel full while depriving our bodies of the essential nutrients required for healthy functioning. When we eat a bland and not nourishing diet, we ultimately allow ourselves to be dumbed down. We need to be thinking correctly, we need to be moving properly, and we are not functioning at our highest possible potential. These things are highly damaging and can lead to poor coordination and depression. On some level, we all know that processed foods are less healthy than the foods we should be consuming regularly. Our bodies know it, even if our minds are not aware. And we suffer for it. We have stress about it. When we indulge in unhealthy foods, whether we are addicted to them or not, our bodies know it. And, whether it's a subconscious occurrence or not, we often punish ourselves. We know that we are doing something wrong. We feel upset about it and dissatisfied, even if we are currently processing it.

Processed foods are also high in artificial colorings that have been proven to be highly carcinogenic. When we are eating foods that have fixed coloring in them, we are essentially swallowing dye. Would you want to eat hair dye? Not really. But these types of chemicals are what is used in your food. They stay in your body and do not come out. They dye your organs on the inside. They are highly dangerous and can lead to cancer. There also full of preservatives. Processed food stays on the shelf for a very long time. Longer than is healthy and normal. Any typical milk bottle would not last for months at a time. It would curdle and spoil. The same as with cheeses, and the same as with other foods that you find on the shelves that have long shelf lives. Shelf lives are essential for companies to establish because they can make more money if their food can stay on the shelf longer. They will do whatever it takes, whether healthier or not, for the human body to ensure they make the most money possible.

Preservatives often include unhealthy and unnatural chemicals and excessive amounts of salt. Neither of these is good for the body at all. Processed foods can lead to issues with the heart, and hypertension, because of the excessive amount of salt in these foods. High blood pressure is a common occurrence among people who survive off of processed foods, and obesity and heart attacks are some of the number one killers in North America. This has absolutely everything to do with the standard American diet. The sad part is that even if you know it is unhealthy, the chemicals, high sugar, and fat content make these processed foods extremely addicting. The body craves them, which can be almost as dangerous as drug addiction. When you are addicted to food that is neither nourishing nor healthy, it can have long-term consequences on your health and development.

Another way that processed foods contribute to obesity is because we digest them far too quickly compared to foods that are rich in healthy dietary fiber. If we are digesting these foods quickly and they are not filling us up because we are not receiving the fiber that provides us with the whole feeling, we are not even burning the same amount of energy as we would digest healthy foods. This means we eat more and digest less, leading to fast and rapid weight gain. The calories present in your body are much higher when you are on a diet of processed foods. You burn far more calories when eating healthy, whole foods rich in dietary fibers. Unfortunately, this means that people who live and subsist on a diet of processed foods will ultimately gain weight whether they want to or not. And they will provide you with a different amount of energy because they are nourishing. They are likely to leave you tired and sluggish and feeling far too full because you eat a lot more of these unhealthy, sugar-filled foods without feeling content or satiated. Processed food is not appropriately metabolized in our bodies. They are quickly turned to fat. Not only that, but they are high in fat. They are often full of hidden fat and sugars. Vegetable oil is one of the primary ingredients in many of these processed meals, along with high fructose corn syrup, which is a huge culprit in weight gain.

If every processed food on the shelves contained high fructose corn syrup, and most of them do, it is no wonder that North America is facing the worst obesity epidemic in world history. Hydrogenated oils are highly unhealthy because they do not break down. They remain in your body and become merged with the fat cells. These oils make fat far more challenging to burn off. They are harder to get rid of, and that type of stubborn fat can lead to obesity very quickly. The ingredients in processed foods lack most of the nutritional value humans need to function at their highest potential. We need natural food's fibers, vitamins, and minerals before genuinely thriving.

If you can only partially avoid processed foods, you should eat them in moderation. They are dangerous. They can make us feel sluggish, irritable, and unhappy overall. Our dispositions can go from positive to negative when we go from a healthy diet and ultimately find ourselves consumed with nothing but processed foods that are too sugary, fatty, and unhealthy. Our bodies crave nutrition. The most accessible and beneficial thing you can do for yourself is to provide your body with that nutrition. It can be hard to adjust to changing routines, such as subsisting on processed foods, and it can sometimes be very frustrating. You have to spend a lot more time in the kitchen cooking and considering your health and your meals. But ultimately, eating processed foods can kill you and cut you off from yourself. You are consuming toxins and avoiding foods that can act as antioxidants that will give you a chance to get rid of the waste you are putting into your body.

Processed foods are the same as junk foods. They are no different. They are healthier, seemingly junk foods. They are snacks in disguise. To become healthy and to feel healthy, avoiding processed foods at all costs is the first and most effective step that you can take. Don't let yourself be fooled by packaging that claims these foods are healthy. They are saturated, fat, sugar, and salt, lacking in anything nourishing your body. Do everything you can to change your habit of relying on processed foods. Eating healthy is easy and possible if you set your mind to it. Just remember the strategy of walking around the grocery store to pick up the fresh produce and meat as opposed to walking through the aisles full of dangerous and alluring packaging hiding the dangers of the processed food within.

CHAPTER FOURTEEN: COMPLETE MEAL PLANNING

Meal planning can be one of the most critical aspects of developing a healthy lifestyle. When we cannot visualize the future of our eating, it can be effortless to succumb to the temptations of unhealthy foods to become addicted. Especially if it is our habit to eat them rather than eating the foods that will nourish us. Meal planning is quite an endeavor. It can be intimidating, especially to someone who lacks self-organization. If you find yourself having a hard time with meal planning, don't fret. There are many ways that you can begin to delve into meal planning that is fun and easy, whether you struggle with creativity in the kitchen or not.

There are many meal-planning kits that you can buy. Many of them can order boxes full of fresh foods to cook with and include recipes you can use. This can be very helpful if you are not used to cooking, especially when poor eating habits and a busy work schedule make it seem not easy to carve out the time necessary to make full, nourishing meals. The first step in meal planning is research. If you are going to get yourself healthy, you have to look at your options. Researching recipes is the best first place to start.

Accumulating a binder full of healthy foods you want to try out can be fun and educational. It will open your mind to several food possibilities you may have otherwise scoffed at as too complex to prepare or teach you things you had never known.

Recipes can be mind-opening, especially when interested in making new discoveries. Cooking can be a hard habit, but once you begin to master it, you will be surprised by just how much freedom you can find in putting a meal together for yourself that is both health-conscious and delicious! Look at recipe books and magazines and get an accumulation of recipes you want to try. Start with the things that look the most delicious and nourishing, and if you are a novice in the kitchen, look at the things that seem the simplest. Next, keep your recipes organized in a simple way that is easy to navigate. If you find yourself overwhelmed by a lack of organization, it will make meal planning much more difficult. When beginning a new habit, you want to ensure that you are doing everything as simply as possible. Too much change at once can be demanding on your system, and you should always try to implement small, easy changes until they have become a new habit.

Make sure they are easily accessible so that when you want to begin preparing your meal, you can do so easily. If you use a binder, consider laminating the pages or using plastic sleeves so that if you use it in the kitchen, they are not affected by water or other food contamination. When you organize your recipes, it will help to put them in order of breakfast meals, lunch meals, dinner meals, and snacks. This will help you reference the proper recipes more quickly once you start cooking. You could organize your binder by day of the week and have your meals planned out every day and printed out in the binder. There are many ways you could organize your recipes. Do what makes the most sense to you intuitively. Don't force yourself to adhere to an organization that doesn't work for you. Instead, ensure you are doing what works best for you in your own life.

Make sure that you are taking the time to regularly seek out new recipes that stand out to you to keep your creative juices flowing and your kitchen exciting. There are many types of recipes you can try, and the more you attempt, the more interesting going on a journey of healthy eating can be! Next, explore software such as Excel on Microsoft Office that will help you to organize your meal planning. On Excel, you will find a plethora of templates you can choose from to help yourself plan out your meals by day, time, and week. This can be a hugely valuable resource!

If you prefer not to use excel, there are apps you can download on your phone, tablet, or another device to help you better utilize your time and resources. You can even go the old-fashioned route and buy a notebook specially designed for planning meals. This is crucial in ensuring your meals are organized and easily accessible. Having a meal plan is extremely helpful for embarking upon a journey of healthy eating. Creating good habits takes time and patience, and you will inevitably slip somewhere. But that doesn't mean you must stay stuck on the ground! It means you must get back up and keep trying because giving up is far easier than sticking to your plans. One thing that can help with meal planning is sticking with the theme. For example, many people have specific themes like taco Tuesday or another day assigned for a specific type of meal. If that helps you to stay on track, feel free to imitate that type of meal planning. It is done for a reason it works and helps keep things simple and streamlined.

It can be very annoying to find yourself stuck doing a lot of planning and preparation every week or month, so if you want to keep things easy, that can be an excellent way. You could have a theme for biweekly meals, such as taco Tuesday one night and rice and vegetables Tuesday the next, and alternate between them. There is no wrong way to plan your meals. What you have to make sure you do is observe and follow through. Follow-through is necessary for everything else to become redundant and easier. Something that can truly help you to succeed at meal planning is accountability. If you let somebody who knows you and cares about you know that you are attempting to plan your meals, ask them if they would be willing to help you to stick to your routine. They can help you by asking questions about how things are going and whether or not you are staying on track. They may also choose to encourage you and cheer you on through your endeavors. However, if they choose to support you, they can be very rewarding for both of you. If they are a positive and supportive person, it can be great to know that you have people rallied in your corner who genuinely want you to succeed. Just make sure that you are weeding out toxic people who bring you down by turning the attention onto themselves or making you feel it will be difficult for you to accomplish your goals. Sure, constructive feedback can be beneficial, but if you are not seeking constructive feedback, it can, at times, be toxic. Ensure you understand the difference between a toxic person masquerading as supportive and a supportive person who wants to see you thrive.

Another way to take accountability is by taking personal accountability. Personal accountability can be achieved through journaling and self-affirmations. Talking to yourself about your goals, what you do internally or out loud, can be an excellent way to help you stay focused and ask yourself whether or not you are doing the things you hope to accomplish. If you find that you are not, instead of beating yourself up about it, consider your obstacles and move on as you begin to uncover them. The only way you will ever be a failure is if you do not try. If you try, everything will ultimately fall into place because you are making an effort and creating positive changes in your life.

Journaling is helpful for many reasons. They can help you to write down what you have eaten and when and how much. This will give you a good idea of what you can expect from yourself. The things that you are unhappy with, you should address and take note of them. But instead of being angry at yourself for not being a trickle right away, remember that it is a process, and you must go slowly. Instead of implementing a fundamental change in routine and planning out every meal for the next month when you have never done it before, start slow by easing into one or two meals a week, then gradually adding in the rest as you do feel comfortable with the process. Make it something that does not shock your system. Gradual change is the most lasting. And journaling about your experiences will help you uncover your innermost thoughts about the process and things you might not even realize were holding you back. You will begin to sense patterns in your behavior and predict when you might be tempted to get off track and why. If you can identify these trigger points, it will be easier to avoid them in the future. Meal planning can be an exciting endeavor. Even if you don't enjoy that type of organization, it can be gratifying to think about what you will be putting in your body and take the steps necessary to do so. Everybody deserves a chance to become the healthiest and most healthy version of themselves possible. With meal planning and a healthy dose of self-esteem, you will be well on your way to a lifestyle of healthy eating.

CONCLUSION

Healthy eating can be challenging to begin, significantly if you need to develop healthy eating habits from a young age. However, it is possible to become a more health-conscious and proactive person. Fortunately, every day that we wake up living and breathing, we can begin to better ourselves and move forward in our lives. Becoming the best version of ourselves can seem intimidating at first. Still, once you realize that every choice you make impacts your life, whether positive or negative, it becomes a lot easier to see the course of your actions before they come back to haunt us. Poor eating habits are choices that will come back to haunt us. If we are not careful, we will develop health problems later in life because we were not conscientious of what we put into our bodies when we were younger. Healthy eating and exercise is the only way to create a healthy and happy body and mind.

We become stir-crazy and restless when we stay stuck in our homes all day, eating nothing but sugar and fat-laden processed foods and watching TV without exercising. The standard American diet is dangerous and costs people their lives. Don't let yourself become one of those people. Instead, make the choices you need to make to truly better yourself and become the best version of yourself possible. Make choices that will make your family proud and provide them with your presence in their lives for years. When we are not taking care of ourselves, this is very selfish. There are people around us who care deeply for the people we are and the value we bring to their lives, whether we realize it or not. Everybody deserves a chance to take their future into their own hands and create positive changes that will benefit them for years.

Healthy eating is just one of many ways that you can begin to better yourself and prepare your mind and body for the future. Suppose you want to be independent and active for as long as possible without costing yourself thousands of dollars in medical bills and other expenses. In that case, healthy eating is something that you should begin sooner rather than later. If not, it is bound to become a drain on your life, both materially and physically. By reading this book and utilizing the information, you are more prepared to take the first step toward a healthy lifestyle. Planning your meals and becoming more aware of why it is essential to make healthy food choices will drastically improve your quality of life now and for years to come. All you have to do is stick with it, and you will immediately begin to see the positive health effects of healthy eating! All you have to do is try. You can do this!

ABOUT THE AUTHOR

Steven Smith

The author is passionate about nutrition and sharing evidence-based insights on healthy eating. His work promotes wellness and healthy lifestyles for individuals to improve their diets and live healthier lives.

BOOKS BY THIS AUTHOR

Savor The Season: Fresh And Flavorful Recipes For Every Time Of Year

Savor the Season: Fresh and Flavorful Recipes for Every Time of Year is a must-have cookbook for any food lover who appreciates the beauty of cooking with seasonal ingredients. From light and refreshing summer salads to hearty winter stews, this cookbook offers an abundance of delicious and nutritious recipes that are perfect for every season. This cookbook provides a diverse range of dishes that celebrate the unique flavors of each season. From the bright and vibrant fruits and vegetables of summer to the warming spices of fall and winter, Savor the Season offers something for every palate.

In addition to the mouth-watering recipes, this cookbook also provides practical tips and techniques for selecting and storing seasonal produce, as well as guidance on basic cooking techniques to help bring out the best in each ingredient. Whether you're an experienced chef or just starting out in the kitchen, Savor the Season offers something for everyone. With its stunning photography, easy-to-follow recipes, and emphasis on fresh, flavorful ingredients, this cookbook is sure to become a staple in any home kitchen. If you're looking to expand your culinary horizons and savor the flavors of each season, then Savor the Season is the perfect cookbook for you.